BLOOD TYPE B FOOD LIST

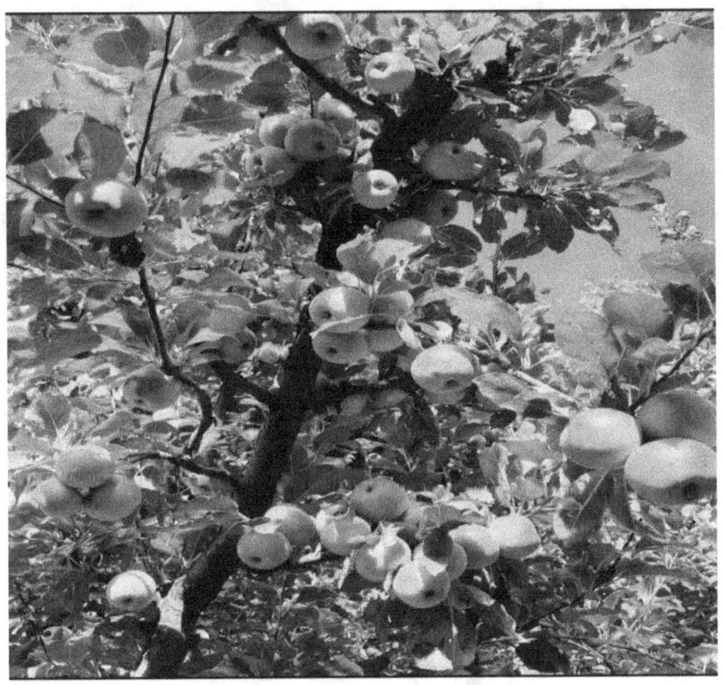

LORENE PEACHEY

DISCLAIMER

The content within this book reflects my thoughts, experiences, and beliefs. It is meant for informational and entertainment purposes. While I have taken great care to provide accurate information, I cannot guarantee the absolute correctness or applicability of the content to every individual or situation. Please consult with relevant professionals for advice specific to your needs.

TO GAIN ACCESS TO MORE BOOK BY THE AUTHOR SCAN THE QR CODE

TABLE OF CONTENTS

INTRODUCTION

In the quiet corridors of my kitchen, amidst the fragrant dance of herbs and the sizzle of wholesome ingredients, I found my calling. A calling that has guided my life's journey, a journey devoted to unraveling the mysteries of dietary needs and concocting recipes that not only tantalize the taste buds but also nurture the very essence of our well-being. Hello, dear readers, I am Lorene Peachey, your culinary companion on a voyage through the fascinating world of blood type-specific nutrition.

It all began years ago when I stumbled upon the profound impact of blood types on our dietary requirements. Little did I know that this revelation would become the cornerstone of my life's work. In my quest for understanding, I immersed myself in the realms of nutritional science, a journey that has spanned decades, filled with countless trials and triumphs.

Why, you may ask, did I dedicate my life to this cause? The answer lies in the transformative power that lies within the food we consume. Our bodies, intricate and unique, respond differently to various nutrients based on our blood types. As a seasoned nutritionist with over 25 years of experience, I have witnessed the profound impact that aligning our diets with our blood types can have on our overall well-being.

Have you ever wondered why a certain diet plan worked wonders for your friend but left you feeling sluggish and discontent? The answer may very well lie in the intricate dance between your blood type and the foods you consume. As I delved deeper into this connection, I couldn't help but ponder – could our dietary choices be the key to unlocking our true potential, both physically and emotionally?

Consider this: What if the secret to your vitality, your energy, and your overall health lay not in generic dietary advice but in a personalized approach tailored to your specific blood type? It's not merely about the food we eat; it's about understanding the language our bodies speak and responding with a symphony of nutrients that resonate with our unique biological composition.

Imagine a world where the simple act of choosing the right foods for your blood type could be the catalyst for a healthier, more vibrant life. A world where you not only savor the flavors but also nourish your body at a cellular level. It's a tantalizing prospect, isn't it? But, my friends, this journey is not just about tantalizing the taste buds; it's about sparking a revolution within, a revolution that transcends the boundaries of mere sustenance.

Now, let me pose a question that might stir the echoes of your own nutritional journey – how often have you felt a lingering fatigue, a sense of imbalance, or perhaps an unexplained discomfort after a meal? What if these signals were your body's way of communicating, urging you to pay attention to the foods that truly harmonize with your blood type?

The consequences of disregarding these signals can be profound. Picture this: indulging in a diet that doesn't align with your blood type is like forcing a square peg into a round hole. It might fit temporarily, but over time, the strain becomes apparent. Digestive woes, low energy levels, and a general sense of malaise may start to creep in, casting a shadow over your daily life.

But fret not, for I bring tidings of a culinary salvation – a meticulously crafted blood type B food list that not only addresses your dietary needs but elevates your entire well-being. This isn't just about restriction; it's about liberation – freeing yourself from the shackles of generic diets and embracing a gastronomic journey that aligns with your unique genetic blueprint.

As we embark on this adventure together, let me assure you that the benefits extend far beyond the realm of mere sustenance. Picture a life where your energy levels soar, your digestion hums like a well-tuned engine, and your mood dances to the rhythm of wholesome nutrients. This, my friends, is the promise of the blood type B food list – a promise backed by years of research, dedication, and a heartfelt desire to see you thrive.

Allow me to share a glimpse of the wonders that await you. The blood type B food list isn't just a collection of ingredients; it's a symphony of flavors designed to complement your unique physiology. From vibrant fruits to lean proteins and nutrient-rich vegetables, each item on this list is handpicked to support your blood type, offering a banquet of benefits for your body and soul.

One might wonder, why the emphasis on tailoring our diets to our blood types? The answer lies in the intricate dance between our blood and the foods we consume. Just as a conductor orchestrates a symphony, our blood type orchestrates the way our bodies respond to various nutrients. By aligning our diets with this inherent rhythm, we unlock a cascade of benefits that extend far beyond the surface.

Consider the advantages of adopting the blood type B food list. It's not merely about avoiding certain foods; it's about embracing a culinary lifestyle that enhances your vitality, supports your immune system, and promotes overall well-being. The foods on this list aren't just fuel; they are elixirs crafted to nourish, rejuvenate, and elevate you to your fullest potential.

Now, let's delve into the perilous realm of ignoring the call of your blood type. Picture a scenario where you consistently consume foods that clash with your physiological makeup. The consequences are not merely physical; they reverberate through the very fabric of your well-being. Digestive discomfort, inflammation, and a weakened immune system may become unwelcome companions on your journey.

But, my dear readers, fear not the dangers that lurk in the shadows, for the blood type B food list is your beacon of light. It's a roadmap to wellness, a guide that empowers you to make choices that resonate with your body's unique language. The risks of straying from this path are not just physical; they extend into the realm of emotional well-being.

Consider this: when your body is nourished and thriving, so too is your mind. The connection between what we consume and how we feel is undeniable. Imagine a life where the fog of fatigue lifts, replaced by mental clarity and a sense of vitality. It's not a mere fantasy; it's the promise of aligning your diet with your blood type, a promise that extends beyond the realm of the physical into the very core of your emotional being.

As we traverse this culinary landscape together, let me share a glimpse of the countless hours spent in my kitchen laboratory. The creation of the blood type B food list wasn't a task; it was a labor of love. Each recipe, each ingredient was carefully chosen, not just for its nutritional profile, but for its ability to harmonize with the unique composition of blood type B.

The beauty of this journey lies not just in the destination but in the exploration itself. It's an invitation to rediscover the joy of eating, the pleasure of savoring every bite knowing that it contributes to your overall well-being. The blood type B food list isn't a restrictive regimen; it's a celebration of culinary diversity, a mosaic of flavors that cater to your body's specific needs.

So, my dear readers, are you ready to embark on a journey of culinary enlightenment? Are you prepared to bid farewell to the one-size-fits-all approach and embrace a diet that aligns with the very essence of who you are? The benefits await you – a renewed sense of energy, improved digestion, and a harmonious balance that extends into every facet of your life.

As we unravel the secrets of the blood type B food list together, let's savor the anticipation of a healthier, more vibrant future. This isn't just a book; it's a companion on your journey to optimal well-being. So, grab your aprons, sharpen your knives, and let's embark on a culinary adventure that transcends the boundaries of ordinary diets and leads you to the extraordinary realm of blood type-specific nutrition. The kitchen awaits, and so does a healthier, happier you.

CHAPTER 1

OVERVIEW OF BLOOD TYPE B

Blood type B is one of the four major blood types determined by the presence or absence of specific antigens on the surface of red blood cells. Individuals with blood type B have B antigens on their red blood cells and anti-A antibodies in their plasma. The ABO blood typing system classifies blood into four types: A, B, AB, and O. Blood type B is characterized by the presence of B antigens and the absence of A antigens.

Overview of Blood Type B:

1. **Genetic Basis:** Blood type is inherited from parents. If both parents carry the B gene, their offspring are likely to have blood type B. The presence of the B gene on one or both chromosomes determines blood type B.

2. **Compatible Blood Types:** Individuals with blood type B can receive blood from donors with blood types B and O. Conversely, they can donate blood to individuals with blood types B and AB. It is crucial for blood transfusions to match blood types to prevent adverse reactions.

3. **Geographical Distribution:** Blood type distributions vary across populations. Blood type B is more prevalent in certain regions, such as parts of Asia and Central Asia. The frequency of blood type B can differ significantly among different ethnic groups.

4. **Medical Considerations:** Blood type B individuals may have specific susceptibilities or resistances to certain diseases. Research is ongoing to explore potential connections between blood type and health conditions, but no definitive conclusions have been reached.

Importance of Blood Type in Diet:

The concept of blood type diets, popularized by Dr. Peter J. D'Adamo in his book "Eat Right 4 Your Type," suggests that an individual's blood type should influence their dietary choices. According to this theory:

1. **Recommended Foods:** People with blood type B are often advised to consume a balanced diet that includes a variety of foods. This may include lean meats, fish, dairy, grains, fruits, and vegetables. The emphasis is on maintaining balance and avoiding excessive consumption of certain food groups.

2. **Foods to Limit or Avoid:** The blood type B diet recommends limiting or avoiding specific foods, such as certain types of meat, dairy, and grains. For example, some versions of the diet suggest that individuals with blood type B should reduce their intake of chicken and replace it with lamb or mutton.

3. **Individual Variations:** It's important to note that individual responses to diets can vary, and there is limited scientific evidence supporting the specific blood type diet recommendations. As with any dietary plan, it is advisable for individuals to consult with healthcare professionals or registered dietitians to ensure nutritional adequacy.

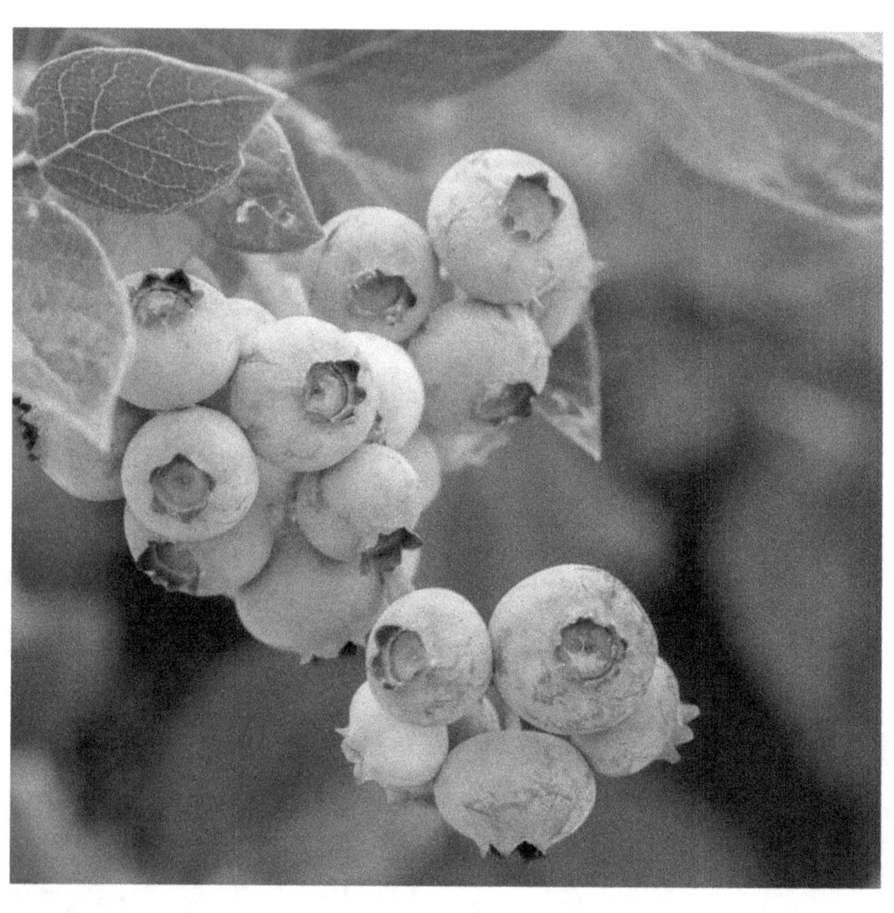

CHAPTER 2

BLOOD TYPE B

CHARACTERISTICS

Physical Traits:

1. **Moderate Build:** Individuals with blood type B are often associated with a moderate or balanced physique. They tend to have a well-proportioned build without extreme characteristics.

2. **Dark Hair and Eyes:** Blood type B individuals may commonly have dark hair and eyes. However, like any generalization, variations exist, and physical traits can be influenced by a combination of genetic factors.

Personality Traits:

1. **Adaptable and Flexible:** Blood type B individuals are often described as flexible and adaptable. They can adjust well to changing circumstances and are open to new experiences.

2. **Creative and Imaginative:** There may be a tendency towards creativity and imagination. Blood type B individuals may have a flair for artistic expression and innovative thinking.

3. **Individualistic:** They are often considered independent and individualistic, valuing their autonomy and freedom. They may prefer to approach tasks and challenges in their own way.

Metabolic Considerations:

1. **Balanced Metabolism:** Blood type B individuals are said to have a balanced metabolic profile. This means they may have the ability to metabolize a variety of foods efficiently.

2. **Tolerance to Dairy:** Some sources suggest that individuals with blood type B may have a better tolerance for dairy products compared to some other blood types.

Exercise Preferences:

1. **Variety in Exercise:** Blood type B individuals are often advised to engage in a variety of exercises. This may include activities that combine both physical and mental components, such as yoga, tai chi, or martial arts.

2. **Moderate Physical Activity:** A balanced approach to exercise is recommended, with a focus on activities that promote overall well-being without the need for extreme or overly strenuous workouts.

Dietary Considerations:

1. **Balanced Diet:** A balanced and varied diet is often recommended for blood type B individuals. This includes a mix of lean meats, fish, dairy, grains, fruits, and vegetables.

2. **Limiting Certain Foods:** Some versions of the blood type B diet suggest limiting certain foods, such as chicken, corn, lentils, and tomatoes. However, it's important to approach dietary recommendations with individual variations in mind.

3. **Emphasis on Lamb and Fish:** Lamb and fish are often recommended as protein sources for blood type B individuals. These foods are believed to be more compatible with their metabolism.

Contact the Author

Thank you for reading my book! I would love to hear from you, whether you have feedback, questions, or just want to share your thoughts. Your feedback means a lot to me and helps me improve as a writer.

Please don't hesitate to reach out to me through

lorenepeachey@gmail.com

I look forward to connecting with my readers and appreciate your support in this literary journey. Your thoughts and comments are valuable to me.

CHAPTER 3

FRUITS

1. **Blueberries:**

    - Nutritional Information (per 1 cup):

        - Calories: 84

        - Carbohydrates: 21 grams

        - Fiber: 3.6 grams

        - Vitamin C: 14.4 mg (24% DV)

        - Antioxidants: Rich in anthocyanins, which have various health benefits.

2. **Papaya:**

    - Nutritional Information (per cup, chunks):

        - Calories: 59

        - Carbohydrates: 15 grams

        - Fiber: 2.5 grams

        - Vitamin C: 88.3 mg (147% DV)

        - Enzymes: Contains papain, aiding digestion.

3. **Pineapple:**

- Nutritional Information (per cup, chunks):

    - Calories: 82

    - Carbohydrates: 22 grams

    - Fiber: 2.3 grams

    - Vitamin C: 78.9 mg (131% DV)

    - Bromelain: Enzyme with anti-inflammatory properties.

4. **Plums:**

- Nutritional Information (per plum):

    - Calories: 30

    - Carbohydrates: 8 grams

    - Fiber: 1 gram

    - Vitamin C: 6.3 mg (11% DV)

    - Antioxidants: Rich in phenolic compounds.

5. **Grapes:**

- Nutritional Information (per cup):

    - Calories: 104

    - Carbohydrates: 27 grams

    - Fiber: 1.4 grams

    - Vitamin C: 1.6 mg (3% DV)

    - Resveratrol: Polyphenol with potential health benefits.

6. **Kiwi:**

- Nutritional Information (per medium-sized kiwi):

    - Calories: 61

    - Carbohydrates: 15 grams

    - Fiber: 2.5 grams

    - Vitamin C: 71.1 mg (118% DV)

    - Vitamin K: 41 mg (52% DV)

7. **Cherries:**

- Nutritional Information (per cup):

    - Calories: 87

    - Carbohydrates: 22 grams

    - Fiber: 3 grams

    - Vitamin C: 7 mg (12% DV)

    - Anthocyanins: Known for anti-inflammatory properties.

8. **Cranberries:**

- Nutritional Information (per cup, raw):

    - Calories: 46

    - Carbohydrates: 12 grams

    - Fiber: 4.6 grams

    - Vitamin C: 13.3 mg (22% DV)

    - Proanthocyanidins: May have urinary tract health benefits.

9. **Mango:**

- Nutritional Information (per cup, sliced):

    - Calories: 107

    - Carbohydrates: 28 grams

    - Fiber: 3 grams

    - Vitamin C: 60.1 mg (100% DV)

    - Vitamin A: 1785 IU (36% DV)

10. **Raspberries:**

- Nutritional Information (per cup):

    - Calories: 64

    - Carbohydrates: 15 grams

    - Fiber: 8 grams

    - Vitamin C: 32.2 mg (54% DV)

    - Manganese: 0.8 mg (41% DV)

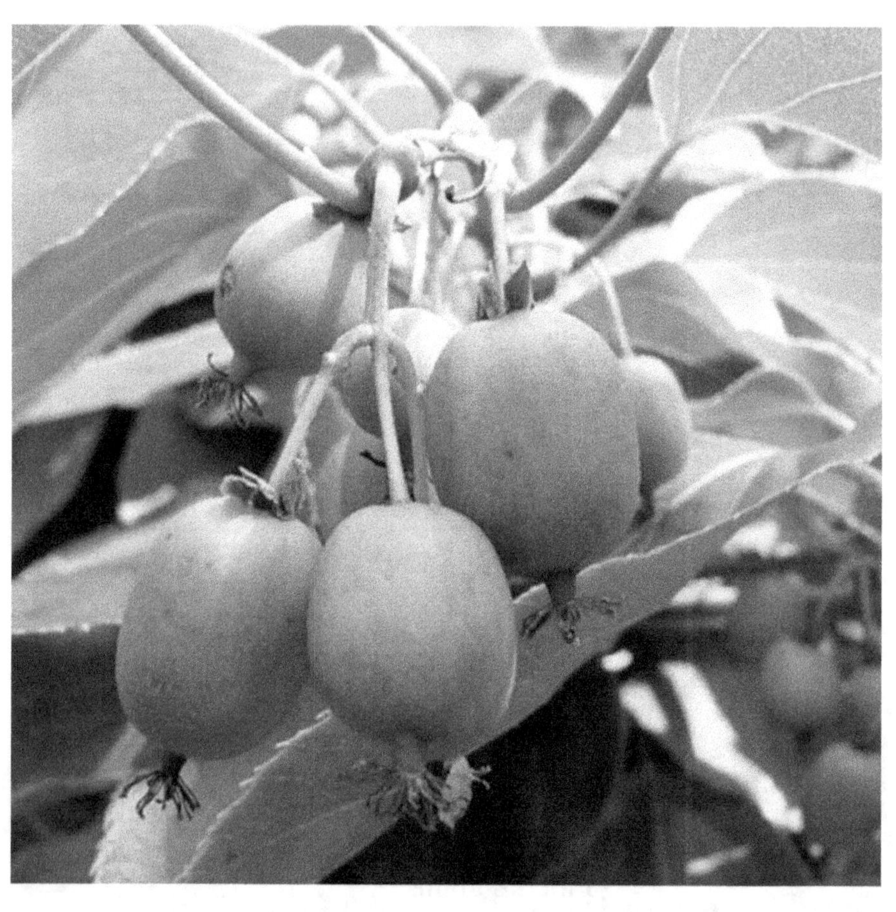

CHAPTER 4
VEGETABLES

1. **Broccoli:**

   - Nutritional Information (per cup, chopped):

     - Calories: 55

     - Carbohydrates: 11 grams

     - Fiber: 5 grams

     - Vitamin C: 135 mg (225% DV)

     - Vitamin K: 220 mcg (276% DV)

2. **Carrots:**

   - Nutritional Information (per medium carrot):

     - Calories: 25

     - Carbohydrates: 6 grams

     - Fiber: 2 grams

     - Vitamin A: 10192 IU (204% DV)

     - Beta-carotene: Important for eye health.

3. **Spinach:**

- Nutritional Information (per cup, cooked):

    - Calories: 41

    - Carbohydrates: 7 grams

    - Fiber: 4 grams

    - Vitamin A: 18856 IU (377% DV)

    - Iron: 6.4 mg (36% DV)

4. **Bell Peppers (Red):**

- Nutritional Information (per cup, sliced):

    - Calories: 46

    - Carbohydrates: 9 grams

    - Fiber: 3 grams

    - Vitamin C: 190 mg (317% DV)

    - Vitamin A: 3726 IU (75% DV)

5. **Cauliflower:**

- Nutritional Information (per cup, chopped):

    - Calories: 27

    - Carbohydrates: 6 grams

    - Fiber: 3 grams

    - Vitamin C: 51.6 mg (86% DV)

    - Vitamin K: 16.6 mcg (21% DV)

6. **Sweet Potatoes:**

- Nutritional Information (per medium sweet potato):

    - Calories: 103

    - Carbohydrates: 24 grams

    - Fiber: 4 grams

    - Vitamin A: 43829 IU (877% DV)

    - Vitamin C: 3.1 mg (5% DV)

7. **Zucchini:**

- Nutritional Information (per cup, sliced):

    - Calories: 20

    - Carbohydrates: 4 grams

    - Fiber: 1 gram

    - Vitamin C: 21 mg (35% DV)

    - Manganese: 0.2 mg (10% DV)

8. **Kale:**

- Nutritional Information (per cup, chopped):

    - Calories: 33

    - Carbohydrates: 6 grams

    - Fiber: 1.3 grams

    - Vitamin A: 10302 IU (206% DV)

    - Vitamin K: 547 mcg (684% DV)

9. **Cabbage:**

- Nutritional Information (per cup, shredded):

    - Calories: 22

    - Carbohydrates: 5 grams

    - Fiber: 2 grams

    - Vitamin C: 28.1 mg (47% DV)

    - Vitamin K: 67.6 mcg (85% DV)

10. **Brussels Sprouts:**

- Nutritional Information (per cup, cooked):

    - Calories: 56

    - Carbohydrates: 12 grams

    - Fiber: 4 grams

    - Vitamin C: 96.7 mg (161% DV)

    - Vitamin K: 218 mcg (273% DV)

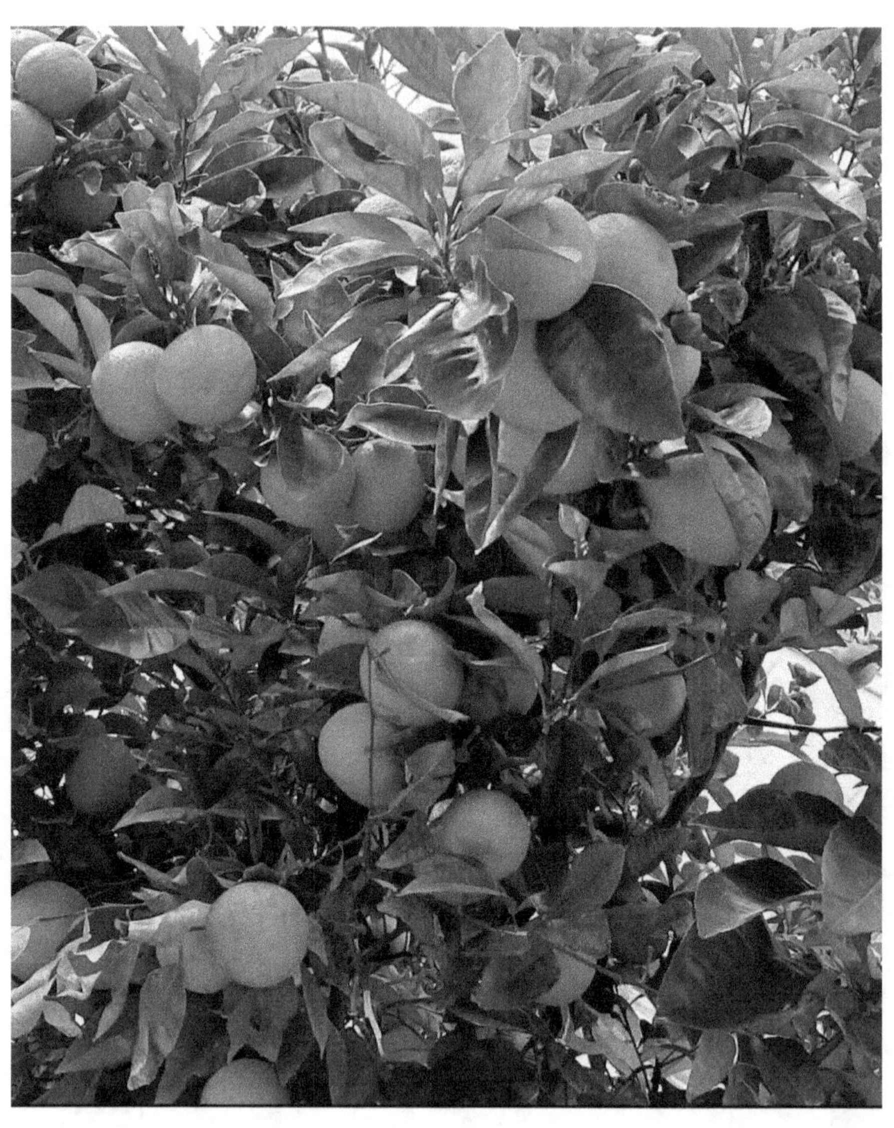

CHAPTER 5

PROTEIN SOURCES

1. **Lamb:**

    - Nutritional Information (per 3 ounces, cooked):

        - Calories: 250

        - Protein: 25 grams

        - Total Fat: 17 grams

        - Iron: 2.3 mg (13% DV)

        - Zinc: 3.3 mg (22% DV)

2. **Salmon:**

    - Nutritional Information (per 3 ounces, cooked):

        - Calories: 206

        - Protein: 22 grams

        - Total Fat: 13 grams

        - Omega-3 Fatty Acids: 1333 mg

        - Vitamin D: 570 IU (95% DV)

3. **Eggs:**

- Nutritional Information (per large egg):

    - Calories: 70

    - Protein: 6 grams

    - Total Fat: 5 grams

    - Choline: 147 mg

    - Vitamin B12: 0.6 mcg (10% DV)

4. **Turkey:**

- Nutritional Information (per 3 ounces, cooked):

    - Calories: 135

    - Protein: 25 grams

    - Total Fat: 3 grams

    - Selenium: 23.8 mcg (34% DV)

    - Vitamin B6: 0.5 mg (23% DV)

5. **Mackerel:**

- Nutritional Information (per 3 ounces, cooked):

  - Calories: 174

  - Protein: 20 grams

  - Total Fat: 10 grams

  - Omega-3 Fatty Acids: 4114 mg

  - Vitamin D: 360 IU (90% DV)

6. **Cottage Cheese:**

- Nutritional Information (per cup, low-fat):

  - Calories: 206

  - Protein: 28 grams

  - Total Fat: 10 grams

  - Calcium: 220 mg (22% DV)

  - Phosphorus: 448 mg (45% DV)

7. **Beef (Lean Cuts):**

- Nutritional Information (per 3 ounces, cooked):

    - Calories: 184

    - Protein: 22 grams

    - Total Fat: 11 grams

    - Iron: 2.1 mg (12% DV)

    - Zinc: 4.5 mg (30% DV)

8. **Quinoa:**

- Nutritional Information (per cup, cooked):

    - Calories: 222

    - Protein: 8 grams

    - Total Fat: 4 grams

    - Fiber: 5 grams

    - Iron: 2.8 mg (15% DV)

9. **Sardines:**

- Nutritional Information (per 3 ounces, canned):

    - Calories: 177

    - Protein: 21 grams

    - Total Fat: 10 grams

    - Omega-3 Fatty Acids: 981 mg

    - Calcium: 382 mg (38% DV)

10. **Tempeh:**

- Nutritional Information (per 3 ounces, cooked):

    - Calories: 140

    - Protein: 16 grams

    - Total Fat: 7 grams

    - Fiber: 4 grams

    - Iron: 2.2 mg (12% DV)

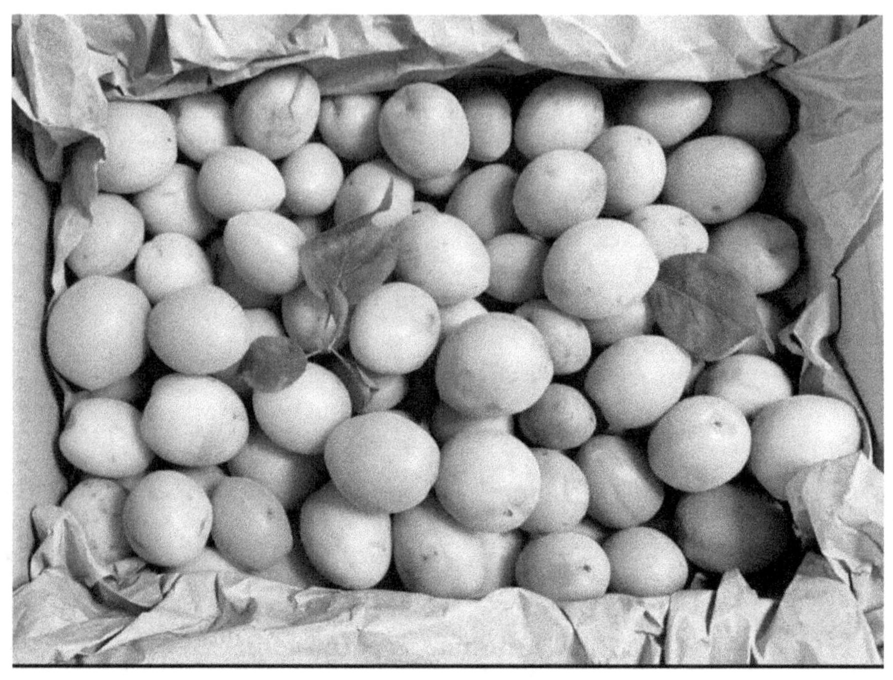

CHAPTER 6

GRAINS

1. **Oats:**

    - Nutritional Information (per 1 cup, cooked):

        - Calories: 147

        - Carbohydrates: 25 grams

        - Fiber: 4 grams

        - Protein: 6 grams

        - Manganese: 1.1 mg (55% DV)

2. **Rice (Basmati):**

    - Nutritional Information (per 1 cup, cooked):

        - Calories: 205

        - Carbohydrates: 45 grams

        - Fiber: 0.6 grams

        - Protein: 4 grams

        - Thiamine: 0.2 mg (15% DV)

3. **Amaranth:**

- Nutritional Information (per 1 cup, cooked):

    - Calories: 251

    - Carbohydrates: 46 grams

    - Fiber: 5 grams

    - Protein: 9 grams

    - Calcium: 116 mg (12% DV)

4. **Barley:**

- Nutritional Information (per 1 cup, cooked):

    - Calories: 193

    - Carbohydrates: 44 grams

    - Fiber: 6 grams

    - Protein: 4 grams

    - Selenium: 19.7 mcg (28% DV)

5. **Millet:**

- Nutritional Information (per 1 cup, cooked):

  - Calories: 207

  - Carbohydrates: 41 grams

  - Fiber: 2 grams

  - Protein: 6 grams

  - Magnesium: 76 mg (19% DV)

6. **Brown Rice:**

- Nutritional Information (per 1 cup, cooked):

  - Calories: 215

  - Carbohydrates: 45 grams

  - Fiber: 3.5 grams

  - Protein: 5 grams

  - Manganese: 1.9 mg (96% DV)

7. **Spelt:**

- Nutritional Information (per 1 cup, cooked):

    - Calories: 246

    - Carbohydrates: 51 grams

    - Fiber: 7.6 grams

    - Protein: 10.7 grams

    - Phosphorus: 178 mg (18% DV)

8. **Wild Rice:**

- Nutritional Information (per 1 cup, cooked):

    - Calories: 166

    - Carbohydrates: 35 grams

    - Fiber: 3 grams

    - Protein: 7 grams

    - Folate: 6 mcg (2% DV)

CHAPTER 7

FOODS TO AVOID OR LIMIT

1. **Chicken:**

   - Nutritional Information (per 3 ounces, cooked):

     - Calories: 165

     - Protein: 25 grams

     - Total Fat: 7 grams

     - Iron: 1.3 mg (7% DV)

     - Phosphorus: 180 mg (18% DV)

2. **Corn:**

   - Nutritional Information (per cup, cooked):

     - Calories: 143

     - Carbohydrates: 31 grams

     - Fiber: 3.5 grams

     - Protein: 5 grams

     - Thiamine: 0.2 mg (15% DV)

3. **Tomatoes:**

- Nutritional Information (per medium tomato):

    - Calories: 22

    - Carbohydrates: 5 grams

    - Fiber: 1.5 grams

    - Vitamin C: 15.6 mg (26% DV)

    - Lycopene: A carotenoid with antioxidant properties.

4. **Wheat:**

- Nutritional Information (per cup, cooked):

    - Calories: 151

    - Carbohydrates: 31 grams

    - Fiber: 4 grams

    - Protein: 6 grams

    - Manganese: 1.9 mg (96% DV)

5. **Peanuts:**

- Nutritional Information (per ounce, dry roasted):

    - Calories: 166

    - Protein: 7 grams

    - Total Fat: 14 grams

    - Fiber: 3 grams

    - Niacin: 4.2 mg (21% DV)

6. **Sesame Seeds:**

- Nutritional Information (per tablespoon, whole):

    - Calories: 52

    - Protein: 1.6 grams

    - Total Fat: 4.5 grams

    - Calcium: 87 mg (9% DV)

    - Iron: 1.3 mg (7% DV)

7. **Buckwheat:**

- Nutritional Information (per 1 cup, cooked):

    - Calories: 155

    - Carbohydrates: 33 grams

    - Fiber: 5 grams

    - Protein: 6 grams

    - Manganese: 1 mg (54% DV)

8. **Lentils:**

- Nutritional Information (per cup, cooked):

    - Calories: 230

    - Carbohydrates: 40 grams

    - Fiber: 15.6 grams

    - Protein: 17.9 grams

    - Folate: 358 mcg (90% DV)

9. **Brazil Nuts:**

- Nutritional Information (per ounce):

    - Calories: 186

    - Protein: 4 grams

    - Total Fat: 19 grams

    - Selenium: 544 mcg (777% DV)

    - Copper: 0.6 mg (31% DV)

10. **Pomegranates:**

- Nutritional Information (per cup, arils):

    - Calories: 83

    - Carbohydrates: 21 grams

    - Fiber: 4 grams

    - Vitamin C: 10.2 mg (17% DV)

    - Antioxidants: Rich in polyphenols.

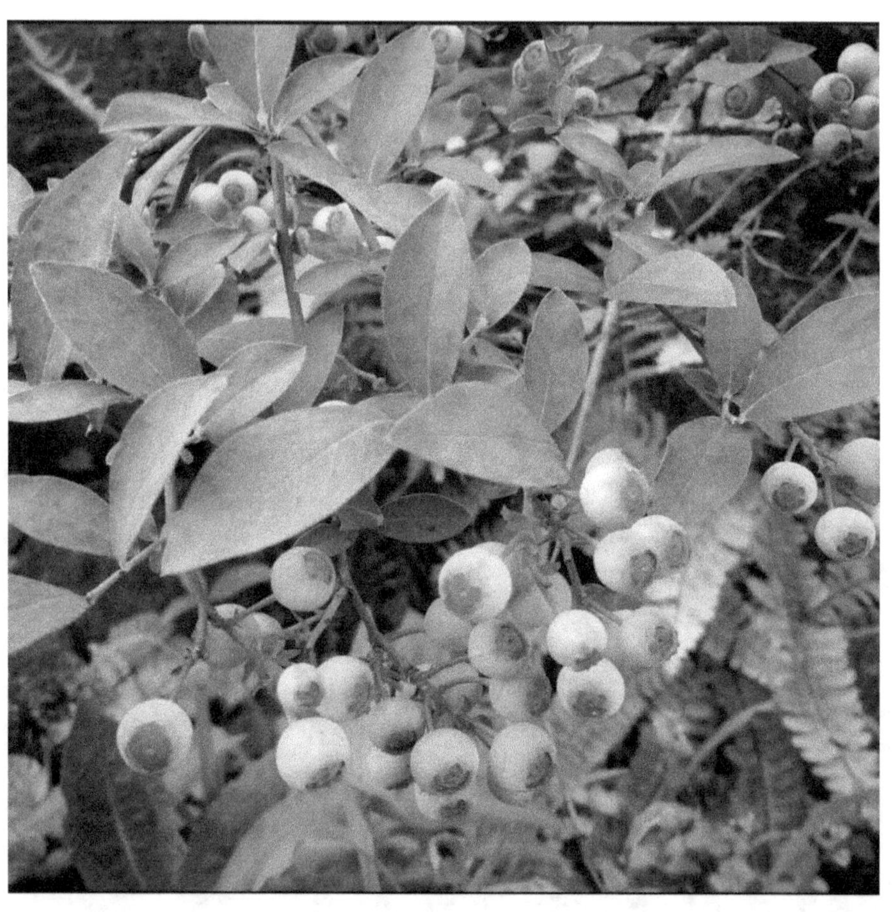

CHAPTER 8

GROCERY SHOPPING GUIDE

1. Plan Your Meals:

- Before heading to the grocery store, plan your meals for the week. Consider your dietary preferences, nutritional needs, and any specific recipes you want to try.

2. Create a Shopping List:

- Based on your meal plan, create a detailed shopping list. Organize it by categories such as fruits, vegetables, proteins, grains, and dairy to make your shopping trip efficient.

3. Choose Fresh Produce:

- Select a variety of fresh fruits and vegetables. Opt for colorful options as they often indicate a range of essential nutrients. Check for freshness, and consider seasonal produce for better flavor and cost savings.

4. Select Lean Proteins:

- Choose lean protein sources such as poultry, fish, tofu, legumes, and lean cuts of meat. Pay attention to the quality and freshness of the proteins you select.

5. Explore Whole Grains:

- Incorporate whole grains like brown rice, quinoa, oats, and whole wheat bread. These provide essential nutrients, fiber, and sustained energy.

6. Include Dairy or Dairy Alternatives:

- Select dairy or dairy alternatives based on your dietary preferences. Choose low-fat or non-fat options for milk, yogurt, and cheese to reduce saturated fat intake.

7. Check Labels:

- Read food labels to understand nutritional content, ingredients, and potential allergens. Look for items with lower added sugars, sodium, and saturated fats.

8. Stock Up on Healthy Fats:

- Include sources of healthy fats such as avocados, nuts, seeds, and olive oil. These fats are beneficial for heart health and overall well-being.

9. Limit Processed Foods:

- Minimize the purchase of heavily processed and pre-packaged foods. These often contain added sugars, preservatives, and high levels of sodium.

10. Stay Hydrated:

- Don't forget to include beverages like water, herbal teas, and, if desired, unsweetened nut milks. Limit sugary drinks and prioritize hydration.

11. Be Mindful of Portions:

- Consider portion sizes to prevent food waste and manage your intake effectively. Buy in bulk when it makes sense, but ensure perishables can be consumed before expiration.

12. Choose Frozen and Canned Options Wisely:

- Opt for frozen or canned fruits and vegetables without added sugars or excessive sodium. These can be convenient and have a longer shelf life.

13. Consider Special Dietary Needs:

- If you have specific dietary requirements or preferences (e.g., gluten-free, vegetarian, or vegan), explore dedicated sections in the store for suitable options.

14. Bring Reusable Bags:

- Bring your reusable bags to reduce plastic waste and contribute to environmental sustainability.

15. Check for Discounts and Sales:

- Take advantage of discounts and sales, but be mindful not to compromise on the nutritional quality of your choices.

CONCLUSION

As we draw the curtains on this culinary odyssey through the enchanting world of blood type B nutrition, I find myself filled with a profound sense of gratitude and excitement. The journey we've embarked upon isn't just about food; it's a testament to the transformative power that lies within the choices we make for our bodies. Together, we've explored the symphony of flavors, danced with the nutrients, and embraced a lifestyle that harmonizes with our blood type.

The blood type B food list is not a mere compilation of ingredients; it's a manifestation of years of research, dedication, and a heartfelt desire to see you thrive. The benefits of aligning your diet with your blood type are not just physical; they extend into the realm of emotional well-being. It's about feeling the vibrancy of life, experiencing the joy of optimal health, and savoring the richness that comes from nourishing your body in harmony with its unique needs.

As you close the pages of this book, my hope is that you carry with you not just recipes and nutritional insights but a newfound appreciation for the intimate connection between your dietary choices and your well-being. The kitchen, once a realm of mere sustenance, now becomes a sanctuary of empowerment, a place where you shape your destiny one meal at a time.

I encourage you to embrace this journey as a lifelong exploration. Experiment with the recipes, savor the flavors, and pay attention to the whispers of your body. Your feedback, dear reader, is not just welcome; it's invaluable. Share your experiences, your culinary triumphs, and even the moments of challenge. Together, we form a community bound by a common goal – the pursuit of a healthier, happier life.

As you step into your kitchen with newfound enthusiasm, remember that this isn't a journey of perfection but one of progress. Celebrate every step, relish every flavor, and honor the unique needs of your body. The blood type B food list is a guide, but you are the maestro, orchestrating the symphony of your well-being.

So, with gratitude in my heart and excitement for the vibrant future that awaits you, I bid you farewell, dear reader. May your culinary adventures be filled with joy, your meals be a source of nourishment, and your journey towards optimal health be nothing short of extraordinary. Here's to a life well-lived, where every bite is a celebration of your unique vitality.

I eagerly await your feedback, your stories, and the shared moments of triumph on this journey. Let's continue this conversation, for it's through our collective experiences that we weave a tapestry of well-being that transcends the pages of this book. Until we meet again in the delightful dance of flavors, be well, be nourished, and savor the extraordinary journey that is your life.

BONUS CHAPTER 1

HEALTHY BLOOD TYPE B

RECIPES

Grilled Salmon with Quinoa Salad:

Cooking Time: 20 minutes

Servings: 4

Ingredients:

- 4 salmon fillets

- 1 cup quinoa, cooked

- 1 cup cherry tomatoes, halved

- 1 cucumber, diced

- 1/4 cup feta cheese, crumbled

- 2 tablespoons olive oil

- Lemon juice, salt, and pepper to taste

Instructions:

1. Season salmon fillets with salt, pepper, and a squeeze of lemon juice.

2. Grill salmon for 4-5 minutes per side.

3. In a bowl, mix cooked quinoa, cherry tomatoes, cucumber, feta, olive oil, and additional lemon juice.

4. Serve grilled salmon over quinoa salad.

Nutritional Information (per serving): Calories: 420 | Protein: 30g | Carbohydrates: 25g | Fat: 22g | Fiber: 4g

Vegetable Stir-Fry with Tofu:

Cooking Time: 15 minutes

Servings: 4

Ingredients:

- 1 block firm tofu, cubed
- 2 cups broccoli florets
- 1 bell pepper, sliced
- 1 carrot, julienned
- 1 cup snow peas
- 3 tablespoons soy sauce
- 1 tablespoon sesame oil
- 2 cloves garlic, minced

Instructions:

1. Press tofu to remove excess water, then stir-fry until golden.

2. Add garlic, broccoli, bell pepper, carrot, and snow peas to the tofu.

3. Stir in soy sauce and sesame oil, cooking until vegetables are tender.

Nutritional Information (per serving): Calories: 280 | Protein: 18g | Carbohydrates: 22g | Fat: 15g | Fiber: 6g

Quinoa and Vegetable Stuffed Peppers:

Cooking Time: 30 minutes

Servings: 6

Ingredients:

- 1 cup quinoa, cooked

- 6 bell peppers, halved and seeds removed

- 1 zucchini, diced

- 1 cup black beans, cooked

- 1 cup corn kernels

- 1 cup diced tomatoes

- 1 teaspoon cumin

- 1 teaspoon chili powder

- Salt and pepper to taste

- Olive oil for drizzling

Instructions:

1. Preheat oven to 375°F (190°C).

2. In a bowl, mix quinoa, zucchini, black beans, corn, diced tomatoes, cumin, chili powder, salt, and pepper.

3. Stuff each bell pepper half with the quinoa mixture.

4. Drizzle with olive oil and bake for 20-25 minutes until peppers are tender.

Nutritional Information (per serving): Calories: 220 | Protein: 8g | Carbohydrates: 40g | Fat: 4g | Fiber: 7g

Spicy Shrimp and Brown Rice Bowl:

Cooking Time: 25 minutes

Servings: 4

Ingredients:

- 1 pound shrimp, peeled and deveined

- 2 cups brown rice, cooked

- 1 bell pepper, sliced

- 1 onion, thinly sliced

- 1 cup snap peas

- 2 tablespoons soy sauce

- 1 tablespoon sriracha

- 1 tablespoon sesame oil

- 2 teaspoons ginger, grated

Instructions:

1. In a wok or skillet, stir-fry shrimp until pink and opaque. Set aside.

2. In the same pan, stir-fry bell pepper, onion, and snap peas until tender-crisp.

3. Add cooked brown rice to the vegetables, then toss in soy sauce, sriracha, sesame oil, and grated ginger.

4. Finally, mix in the cooked shrimp and heat through.

Nutritional Information (per serving): Calories: 320 | Protein: 28g | Carbohydrates: 42g | Fat: 6g | Fiber: 5g

Turkey and Vegetable Skewers:

Cooking Time: 20 minutes

Servings: 4

Ingredients:

- 1 pound turkey breast, cut into cubes
- 1 zucchini, sliced
- 1 red onion, cut into chunks
- 1 bell pepper, cut into squares
- 2 tablespoons olive oil
- 1 teaspoon dried oregano
- 1 teaspoon smoked paprika

Instructions:

1. Preheat the grill or oven.

2. Thread turkey, zucchini, red onion, and bell pepper onto skewers.

3. Mix olive oil, dried oregano, smoked paprika, salt, and pepper. Brush onto skewers.

4. Grill or bake for 10-15 minutes, turning occasionally, until turkey is cooked.

Nutritional Information (per serving): Calories: 280 | Protein: 30g | Carbohydrates: 8g | Fat: 14g | Fiber: 2g

Eggplant and Chickpea Curry:

Cooking Time: 30 minutes

Servings: 4

Ingredients:

- 1 large eggplant, diced

- 1 can (15 oz) chickpeas, drained

- 1 onion, chopped

- 2 tomatoes, diced

- 3 cloves garlic, minced

- 1 tablespoon curry powder

- 1 teaspoon cumin

- 1 teaspoon turmeric

- 1 cup coconut milk

- Fresh cilantro for garnish

Instructions:

1. Sauté onions and garlic until softened. Add diced eggplant and cook until golden.

2. Stir in curry powder, cumin, and turmeric. Add tomatoes and chickpeas.

3. Pour in coconut milk and simmer for 15-20 minutes until flavors meld.

4. Garnish with fresh cilantro before serving.

Nutritional Information (per serving): Calories: 320 | Protein: 10g | Carbohydrates: 38g | Fat: 16g | Fiber: 12g

Sweet Potato and Black Bean Tacos:

Cooking Time: 25 minutes

Servings: 4

Ingredients:

- 2 large sweet potatoes, diced

- 1 can (15 oz) black beans, rinsed and drained

- 1 red onion, finely chopped

- 1 avocado, sliced

- 8 small corn tortillas

- 1 teaspoon cumin

- 1 teaspoon chili powder

- 1 lime, juiced

- Fresh cilantro for garnish

Instructions:

1. Roast sweet potatoes with cumin and chili powder until tender.

2. In a bowl, mix black beans, red onion, and lime juice.

3. Fill corn tortillas with roasted sweet potatoes, black bean mixture, and avocado slices.

4. Garnish with fresh cilantro.

Nutritional Information (per serving): Calories: 290 | Protein: 9g | Carbohydrates: 49g | Fat: 8g | Fiber: 11g

Berry and Spinach Salad with Grilled Chicken:

Cooking Time: 20 minutes

Servings: 2

Ingredients:

- 2 boneless, skinless chicken breasts

- 4 cups baby spinach

- 1 cup mixed berries (strawberries, blueberries, raspberries)

- 1/4 cup feta cheese, crumbled

- 1/4 cup walnuts, chopped

- Balsamic vinaigrette dressing

Instructions:

1. Grill chicken breasts until cooked through.

2. In a large bowl, toss baby spinach with mixed berries, feta, and walnuts.

3. Slice grilled chicken and place on top of the salad.

4. Drizzle with balsamic vinaigrette dressing before serving.

Nutritional Information (per serving): Calories: 350 | Protein: 30g | Carbohydrates: 18g | Fat: 18g | Fiber: 6g

Mediterranean Quinoa Bowl:

Cooking Time: 25 minutes

Servings: 4

Ingredients:

- 1 cup quinoa, cooked

- 1 cup cherry tomatoes, halved

- 1 cucumber, diced

- 1/2 red onion, finely chopped

- 1 cup Kalamata olives, pitted and sliced

- 1 cup feta cheese, crumbled

- 1/4 cup fresh parsley, chopped

- 3 tablespoons olive oil

- 1 lemon, juiced

- Salt and pepper to taste

Instructions:

1. In a large bowl, combine cooked quinoa, cherry tomatoes, cucumber, red onion, olives, feta, and fresh parsley.

2. In a small bowl, whisk together olive oil, lemon juice, salt, and pepper to create the dressing.

3. Pour the dressing over the quinoa mixture and toss until well combined.

4. Serve in bowls, garnished with additional parsley if desired.

Nutritional Information (per serving): Calories: 380 | Protein: 12g | Carbohydrates: 35g | Fat: 22g | Fiber: 6g

Teriyaki Tofu Stir-Fry:

Cooking Time: 20 minutes

Servings: 4

Ingredients:

- 1 block extra-firm tofu, pressed and cubed

- 1 cup broccoli florets

- 1 bell pepper, sliced

- 1 carrot, julienned

- 1 cup snap peas

- 1/2 cup teriyaki sauce

- 2 tablespoons sesame oil

- 3 cloves garlic, minced

- 1 tablespoon ginger, grated

- Green onions and sesame seeds for garnish

Instructions:

1. In a wok or skillet, heat sesame oil over medium-high heat.

2. Add tofu cubes and stir-fry until golden brown. Remove tofu from the pan and set aside.

3. In the same pan, sauté garlic and ginger until fragrant.

4. Add broccoli, bell pepper, carrot, and snap peas. Stir-fry until vegetables are tender-crisp.

5. Return the tofu to the pan, pour in teriyaki sauce, and toss to coat.

6. Garnish with green onions and sesame seeds before serving.

Nutritional Information (per serving): Calories: 280 | Protein: 14g | Carbohydrates: 28g | Fat: 14g | Fiber: 5g

IF YOU WANT MORE RECIPES, YOU CAN CHECK OUT OTHER BOOKS BY THE AUTHOR

GLUTEN-FREE COOKBOOK FOR VEGAN

GLUTEN-FREE COOKBOOK FOR BEGINNERS

GLUTEN-FREE COOKBOOK FOR KIDS

MEDITERRANEAN INSTANT POT COOKBOOK FOR WOMEN

LOW SODIUM SLOW COOKER COOKBOOK

TO GET ACCESS TO MORE BOOKS BY THE AUTHOR SCAN THE QR CODE

BONUS CHAPTER 2
EXERCISE RECOMMENDATION

Individuals with blood type B are often encouraged to engage in a variety of physical activities that promote balance and flexibility. Here are exercise recommendations tailored for blood type B:

1. Moderate Cardiovascular Exercise:

- Engage in moderate-intensity cardiovascular exercises such as brisk walking, cycling, or swimming. Aim for at least 30 minutes on most days of the week to enhance heart health and overall fitness.

2. Variety in Workouts:

- Blood type B individuals tend to benefit from diverse workout routines. Incorporate activities like dance, hiking, or recreational sports to keep workouts interesting and maintain motivation.

3. Yoga and Tai Chi:

- Explore mind-body exercises like yoga and tai chi, which emphasize flexibility, balance, and relaxation. These activities can help manage stress, which is particularly beneficial for blood type B individuals.

4. Strength Training:

- Include strength training exercises using body weight, resistance bands, or free weights. Focus on full-body workouts to build and maintain lean muscle mass.

5. Interval Training:

- Consider incorporating interval training into your routine. This involves alternating between short bursts of high-intensity exercise and periods of lower intensity or rest, promoting cardiovascular fitness.

6. Mindful Exercise Practices:

- Engage in exercises that promote mindfulness, such as Pilates or qigong. These activities help cultivate mental clarity and focus while enhancing physical well-being.

7. Avoid Overtraining:

- Blood type B individuals may benefit from avoiding excessive or intense exercise sessions, as this can lead to stress and fatigue. Listen to your body and allow for adequate recovery.

8. Outdoor Activities:

- Take advantage of outdoor activities that align with your interests, such as hiking, biking, or playing sports. Being in nature can contribute to overall well-being.

9. Consistency is Key:

- Establish a consistent exercise routine that includes a mix of cardiovascular, strength, and flexibility exercises. Consistency is essential for long-term health benefits.

10. Consultation with Fitness Professionals:

- Consider seeking guidance from fitness professionals or personal trainers who can tailor workout plans to your specific needs and fitness goals.